THE GASTRITIS HEALING COOKBOOK FOR BEGINNERS

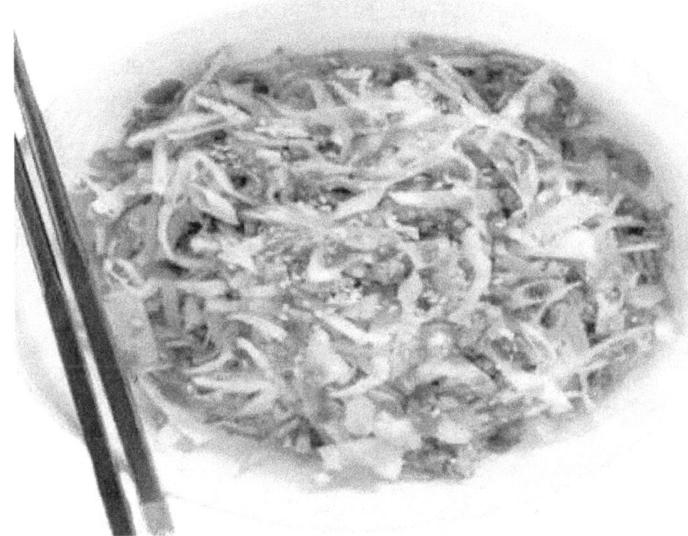

60+ Easy And Delicious Gastritis-Friendly Recipes For Newly Diagnosed To Heal The Immune System And Restore Your Stomach Health

Katherine J. Filer

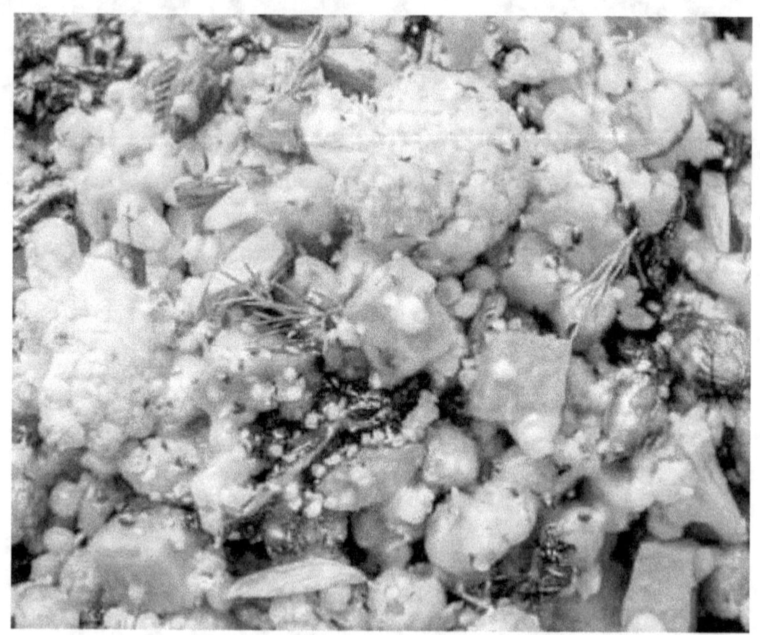

Table of Contents

INTRODUCTION

In the quiet moments before dawn, Margaret sat in her kitchen, sipping her herbal tea, a faint ache gnawing at her stomach. Her journey with gastritis began unexpectedly, disrupting her life in ways she never imagined. A passionate food enthusiast, she cherished the joy of experimenting with diverse cuisines. But her relentless stomach discomfort slowly extinguished that joy.

With a heavy heart, she navigated endless visits to doctors and consumed numerous medications, hoping for relief. However, it wasn't until she stumbled upon the transformative power of food that the tide began to turn. A chance encounter with an ancient healing practice during her travels abroad introduced her to a tantalizing world of gastritis-centric nutrition.

As she embraced this newfound path, she discovered that every ingredient in her kitchen possessed the potential to heal. Through dedicated research, trial, and error, she crafted meals that not only alleviated her gastritis symptoms but also ignited a passion within her to share this knowledge with others.

Margaret's journey from pain to empowerment became the foundation of this book. It's a testament to the extraordinary ability of food to heal and rejuvenate. Within these pages lie not just recipes but a roadmap to wellness, a guide to embracing food as medicine, and a testament to the transformative power of choice.

This book isn't just about healing gastritis; it's a celebration of nourishment, a tribute to the symbiotic relationship between food and health, and an invitation for all to embark on a journey towards vibrant well-being.

Join me as we explore the realms of healing foods, embark on a culinary adventure, and discover the incredible potential of the Gastritis Healing Cookbook.

CHAPTER 1

UNDERSTANDING GASTRITIS

What is Gastritis?

Gastritis refers to the inflammation, irritation, or erosion of the stomach lining. This condition can manifest in various forms, causing discomfort and potentially leading to more severe complications if left unaddressed. The inflammation can be acute, occurring suddenly and temporarily, or chronic, persisting over an extended period.

Types and Variations of Gastritis

1. Acute Gastritis: Typically arises suddenly and is often associated with factors like excessive alcohol consumption, certain medications, bacterial infections (especially Helicobacter pylori), or stress.

2. Chronic Gastritis: This type develops gradually and tends to persist for an extended duration. Chronic gastritis may result from ongoing irritation due to Helicobacter pylori infection, autoimmune conditions, long-term use of nonsteroidal anti-inflammatory drugs (NSAIDs), or other underlying health issues.

3. Erosive Gastritis: Involves the erosion of the stomach lining, leading to ulcers or bleeding. This can be a severe form of gastritis, causing more pronounced symptoms and requiring immediate medical attention.

Symptoms and Signs of Gastritis

1. Abdominal Pain: Discomfort or a burning sensation in the upper abdomen.

2. Nausea and Vomiting: Feelings of queasiness and occasional vomiting may occur.

3. Indigestion: Difficulty in digesting food, often resulting in bloating, belching, or a feeling of fullness.

4. Loss of Appetite: A decreased desire to eat, often accompanied by a feeling of early satiety.

5. Hematemesis or Bloody Stools: Severe cases of gastritis may lead to vomiting blood (hematemesis) or passing bloody stools.

6. Heartburn: A burning sensation in the chest due to stomach acid refluxing into the esophagus.

7. Hiccups: Occasional persistent hiccups might be a sign of gastritis, especially if accompanied by other symptoms.

8. Unexplained Weight Loss: Chronic gastritis can sometimes lead to unexplained weight loss due to decreased appetite and nutrient absorption issues.

9. Fatigue: Feeling tired or weak, often as a result of anemia due to bleeding caused by erosive gastritis.

10. Frequent Bloating or Gas: Experiencing frequent bloating, gas, or discomfort after meals.

Common Causes of Gastritis

1. Helicobacter pylori (H. pylori) Infection: This bacteria is a major cause of gastritis. It infects the stomach lining, causing inflammation and irritation. H. pylori is usually contracted through contaminated food, water, or close contact with an infected person.

2. Regular Use of Nonsteroidal Anti-inflammatory Drugs (NSAIDs): Prolonged use of medications like aspirin, ibuprofen, naproxen, and others can irritate the stomach lining, leading to gastritis. These drugs inhibit enzymes that help protect the stomach lining, increasing vulnerability to inflammation.

3. Excessive Alcohol Consumption: Alcohol can irritate and damage the stomach lining, leading to inflammation and the development of gastritis. Chronic alcohol use increases the risk of this condition.

4. Bile Reflux: When bile flows back into the stomach from the small intestine, it can cause irritation and inflammation of the stomach lining, leading to gastritis. This reflux can occur due to various conditions affecting the digestive system.

5. Smoking: Cigarette smoking can weaken the protective lining of the stomach, making it more susceptible to inflammation and damage, thereby contributing to gastritis.

6. Autoimmune Disorders: In some cases, the body's immune system mistakenly attacks the cells of the stomach lining, leading to chronic inflammation and gastritis. Conditions like autoimmune gastritis result from this immune response.

7. Stress: While stress itself might not directly cause gastritis, it can worsen existing symptoms. High stress levels can amplify stomach discomfort and may contribute to the development of gastritis in susceptible individuals.

8. Pernicious Anemia: This condition occurs when the body lacks intrinsic factor, a protein necessary for absorbing vitamin B12. Without sufficient B12, the stomach lining can become inflamed, leading to a type of gastritis known as autoimmune gastritis.

9. Radiation Therapy or Chronic Illness: Gastritis can also develop as a side effect of radiation therapy targeting the abdominal area. Additionally, chronic illnesses or severe infections can weaken the immune system, making the stomach more susceptible to inflammation and gastritis.

10. Older Age: As people age, the stomach lining tends to become thinner, making it more susceptible to damage and inflammation. This age-related change increases the likelihood of developing gastritis.

Preventive Measures of Gastritis

1. Dietary Modifications: Adopting a healthy diet can significantly aid in preventing gastritis. Avoiding spicy, acidic, or greasy foods that might irritate the stomach lining is essential. Opt for a balanced diet rich in fruits, vegetables, whole grains, and lean proteins to promote overall stomach health.

2. Limiting NSAIDs and Alcohol: Minimize the use of nonsteroidal anti-inflammatory drugs (NSAIDs) like aspirin, ibuprofen, or naproxen, as these medications can irritate the stomach lining and contribute to gastritis. Similarly, limit alcohol consumption or avoid excessive alcohol intake, as it can irritate and damage the stomach lining.

3. Stress Management: Chronic stress can exacerbate gastritis symptoms. Employ stress-reduction techniques such as meditation, yoga, regular exercise, deep breathing exercises, or engaging in hobbies to manage stress levels effectively.

4. Treatment of H. pylori: If diagnosed with an H. pylori infection, it's crucial to seek treatment prescribed by a healthcare professional to eradicate the bacteria. Treating the infection can prevent the development of chronic gastritis associated with H. pylori.

5. Quitting Smoking: Smoking weakens the protective lining of the stomach, making it more susceptible to inflammation and damage. Quitting smoking can significantly reduce the risk of developing gastritis.

6. Careful Medication Use: Follow prescribed dosages for medications, and if possible, consult a healthcare provider before using NSAIDs regularly. Properly managing medications can prevent unnecessary irritation to the stomach lining.

7. Regular Health Check-ups: Periodic health check-ups with a healthcare professional can help detect and manage gastritis or any underlying conditions early. Discuss any recurring symptoms or concerns regarding stomach health during these check-ups.

Foods to Embrace and Avoid

Foods to Eat:

1. High-Fiber Foods: Opt for whole grains like brown rice, oats, and quinoa. These provide essential nutrients and fiber that aid in digestion without irritating the stomach lining.

2. Lean Proteins: Include lean sources of protein like skinless poultry, fish, tofu, and legumes. These are easier to digest and less likely to cause irritation.

3. Fruits: Choose non-acidic fruits such as bananas, melons, apples, and pears. These fruits are gentle on the stomach and provide vitamins and antioxidants.

4. Vegetables: Consume cooked or steamed vegetables like spinach, carrots, green beans, and sweet potatoes. Avoid raw vegetables as they can be harder to digest.

5. Healthy Fats: Incorporate foods rich in healthy fats like avocados, nuts, seeds, and olive oil. These fats are beneficial for overall health and less likely to cause stomach irritation.

6. Probiotic-Rich Foods: Include yogurt with live cultures, kefir, or fermented foods like kimchi and sauerkraut. These help maintain a healthy balance of gut bacteria, aiding digestion.

7. Herbal Teas: Chamomile, ginger, and licorice root teas have soothing properties that can help alleviate gastritis symptoms.

Foods to Avoid:

1. Spicy Foods: Limit or avoid spicy dishes as they can aggravate the stomach lining, causing discomfort and inflammation.

2. Acidic Foods: Citrus fruits, tomatoes, and their derivatives (such as citrus juices or tomato-based sauces) can trigger irritation due to their acidity.

3. High-Fat Foods: Avoid fried foods, fatty cuts of meat, and full-fat dairy products, as they can increase stomach acid production and worsen symptoms.

4. Caffeine: Cut down on caffeinated beverages like coffee, tea, and soda, as they can increase stomach acid and irritation.

5. Alcohol: Minimize or eliminate alcohol consumption, as it can irritate the stomach lining and exacerbate gastritis symptoms.

6. Carbonated Beverages: Avoid carbonated drinks as they can cause bloating and discomfort.

7. Processed and Spicy Condiments: Stay away from hot sauces, chili flakes, and heavily processed condiments, as they can irritate the stomach lining.

Eating Habits

- **Small, Frequent Meals:** Opt for smaller, more frequent meals to ease digestion and prevent overloading the stomach.
- **Chew Thoroughly:** Chew food slowly and thoroughly to aid digestion and reduce stress on the stomach.
- **Hydration:** Drink plenty of water throughout the day to maintain hydration and support proper digestion.

Core Benefits of Following a Gastritis Healing Diet for Beginners

1. Reduced Inflammation: A gastritis healing diet focuses on foods that are gentle on the stomach lining, reducing irritation and inflammation. It helps to alleviate discomfort and pain associated with gastritis.

2. Alleviation of Symptoms: Following this diet can help in alleviating common symptoms of gastritis such as nausea, abdominal pain, bloating, and indigestion. Choosing foods that soothe the stomach promotes overall comfort.

3. Promotion of Healing: A gastritis healing diet emphasizes foods that support the healing process of the stomach lining. Nutrient-rich foods aid in repairing damaged tissues, aiding the stomach in its recovery.

4. Improved Digestion: Opting for easily digestible foods such as lean proteins, whole grains, and cooked vegetables assists in smoother digestion, reducing the workload on the stomach and promoting overall digestive health.

5. Balanced Nutrition: This diet encourages a well-rounded intake of nutrients essential for overall health. It includes a variety of fruits, vegetables, lean proteins, and healthy fats, ensuring adequate nutrition while managing gastritis.

6. Gut Health Support: Incorporating probiotic-rich foods in the diet fosters a healthy balance of gut bacteria. This supports digestive health and aids in reducing inflammation within the digestive tract.

7. Weight Management: By focusing on whole, nutrient-dense foods and avoiding triggers like high-fat or processed items, a gastritis healing diet can contribute to weight management and overall well-being.

8. Stress Reduction: Adopting a specific diet for gastritis can also indirectly alleviate stress associated with managing the condition. Knowing what foods to eat and avoid can provide a sense of control over symptoms.

9. Improved Overall Health: The gastritis healing diet emphasizes consuming foods that are not only gentle on the stomach but also beneficial for overall health. This can lead to improvements in energy levels, mood, and general wellness.

10. Prevention of Complications: By managing gastritis through a healing diet, individuals may reduce the risk of complications associated with chronic inflammation of the stomach lining, such as ulcers or bleeding.

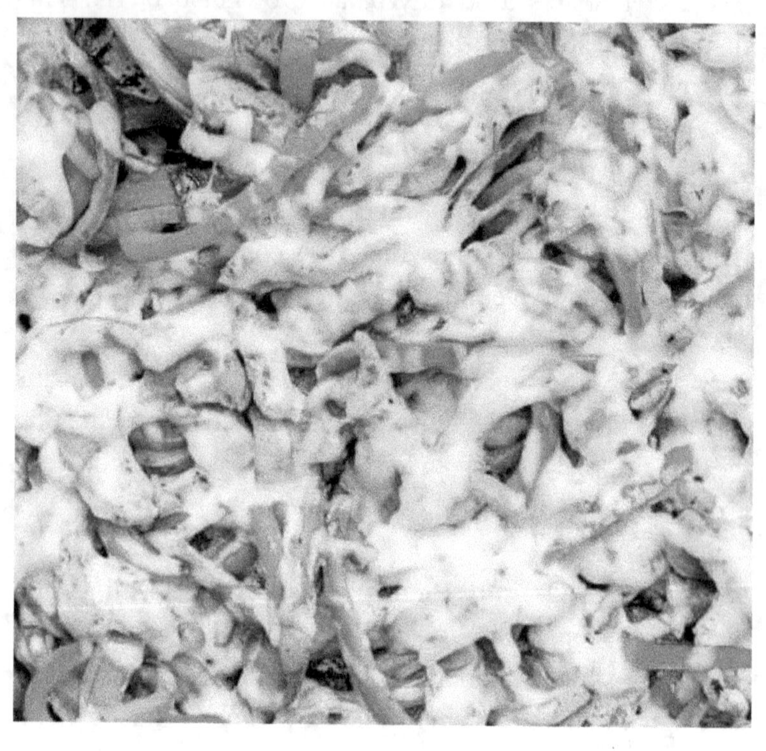

CHAPTER 2

How to Follow a Gastritis Disease Diet

1. Understand the Diet:

- Educate Yourself: Learn about foods that are beneficial and harmful to gastritis. Understand which foods soothe the stomach and which ones can trigger symptoms.

2. Plan Your Meals:

- Create a Meal Plan: Plan meals that include gentle, easily digestible foods. Aim for a variety of fruits, vegetables, lean proteins, and whole grains while avoiding triggers like spicy or acidic foods.

3. Choose Gastritis-Friendly Foods:

- Include Complex Carbohydrates: Opt for whole grains like brown rice, oats, and quinoa as they are gentle on the stomach and provide essential nutrients.

- Lean Proteins: Incorporate lean protein sources such as skinless poultry, fish, tofu, and legumes as they are easier to digest.

- Non-Acidic Fruits: Choose fruits like bananas, melons, apples, and pears, which are less likely to cause irritation due to their low acidity.

- Cooked or Steamed Vegetables: Include cooked or steamed vegetables like spinach, carrots, green beans, and sweet potatoes, as they are easier to digest compared to raw vegetables.

- Healthy Fats: Include sources of healthy fats like avocados, nuts, seeds, and olive oil for their beneficial effects on stomach health.

- Probiotic Foods: Incorporate yogurt with live cultures, kefir, and fermented foods like kimchi and sauerkraut to promote a healthy gut micro biome.

4. Avoid Trigger Foods:

- Spicy Foods: Limit or avoid spicy dishes as they can irritate the stomach lining and worsen gastritis symptoms.

- Acidic Foods: Avoid citrus fruits, tomatoes, and their derivatives, as they can trigger irritation due to their acidity.

- High-Fat Foods: Steer clear of fried foods, fatty cuts of meat, and full-fat dairy products, as they can increase stomach acid production and worsen symptoms.

- Caffeine and Alcohol: Reduce or eliminate caffeinated beverages and alcohol, as they can aggravate gastritis symptoms.

5. Practice Healthy Eating Habits:

- Small, Frequent Meals: Opt for smaller, more frequent meals throughout the day to ease digestion and prevent overloading the stomach.

- Chew Thoroughly: Chew food slowly and thoroughly to aid digestion and reduce stress on the stomach.

6. Hydration:

- Stay Hydrated: Drink plenty of water throughout the day to maintain hydration and support proper digestion.

7. Monitor and Adjust:

- Keep Track: Monitor how your body responds to different foods and adjust your diet accordingly. Note any triggers that worsen symptoms and avoid them.

- Consult a Professional: Seek guidance from a healthcare professional or a registered dietitian to create a personalized diet plan that suits your specific needs and health condition.

Healthy Shopping Ingredients or lists for a Gastritis disease diet

Fruits:

1. Bananas: Low in acidity and gentle on the stomach, providing essential nutrients and fiber.
2. Melons (e.g., Cantaloupe, Honeydew): Non-acidic fruits rich in vitamins and hydration.
3. Apples: Low acidity and a good source of fiber and antioxidants.
4. Pears: Non-acidic fruits with a high fiber content, aiding digestion.

Vegetables:

5. Spinach: Cooked spinach is easy to digest and rich in vitamins and minerals.
6. Carrots: Cooked or grated carrots provide nutrients without causing stomach irritation.
7. Green Beans: Light and easily digestible vegetables suitable for a gastritis diet.
8. Sweet Potatoes: Cooked sweet potatoes offer nutrients and are gentle on the stomach.

Grains:

9. Brown Rice: Whole grain rice that is gentle on the stomach and a good source of fiber.
10. Oats: Easily digestible and a great source of soluble fiber for digestive health.
11. Quinoa: Nutrient-dense, gluten-free grain providing protein and fiber.

Proteins:

12. Skinless Poultry: Lean meats like chicken or turkey breasts are easily digestible.
13. Fish: Non-fatty fish such as salmon or cod are rich in omega-3s and protein.
14. Tofu: Plant-based protein source that's gentle on the stomach.

Dairy:

15. Low-Fat Yogurt: Probiotic-rich yogurt with live cultures for gut health.
16. Kefir: Fermented dairy drink similar to yogurt, beneficial for digestion.

Healthy Fats:

17. Avocados: Rich in healthy fats, vitamins, and minerals that support stomach health.

18. Nuts (e.g., Almonds, Walnuts): Provide healthy fats and are a good source of protein.
19. Seeds (e.g., Chia Seeds, Flaxseeds): Rich in omega-3 fatty acids and fiber.

Others:

20. Ginger: Fresh or ground ginger can soothe the stomach and aid digestion.

When shopping for a gastritis disease diet, prioritize these ingredients to create meals that are gentle on the stomach, provide essential nutrients, and promote digestive health. Incorporating a variety of these items into your diet can help manage gastritis symptoms and support the healing process of the stomach lining. Additionally, it's crucial to avoid foods that trigger irritation or inflammation based on individual sensitivities.

The complications of gastritis disease if the right diet isn't adopted

1. Peptic Ulcers: Chronic inflammation of the stomach lining due to untreated gastritis can lead to the development of peptic ulcers. These are sores that form on the lining of the stomach, esophagus, or small intestine, causing pain, bleeding, and potentially serious complications if left untreated.

2. Bleeding: Severe inflammation caused by untreated gastritis can lead to erosion of the stomach lining, resulting in bleeding. This can manifest as blood in vomit or stool, leading to anemia (low red blood cell count) and requiring medical attention.

3. Anemia: Chronic bleeding from the stomach due to gastritis can result in anemia, characterized by low levels of red blood cells. Anemia can cause fatigue, weakness, and shortness of breath.

4. Increased Risk of Stomach Cancer: Long-term inflammation of the stomach lining, especially when caused by Helicobacter pylori (H. pylori) infection, can increase the risk of developing stomach (gastric) cancer if left untreated for an extended period.

5. Gastroparesis: Chronic inflammation in the stomach can affect its ability to function properly, leading to gastroparesis, a condition where the stomach muscles weaken, causing delayed emptying of food into the small intestine. This can result in bloating, nausea, vomiting, and problems with digestion.

6. Perforation: In severe cases, chronic gastritis left unmanaged can weaken the stomach lining to the point of perforation or rupture, allowing stomach contents to leak into the abdominal cavity. This is a medical emergency requiring immediate surgical intervention.

7. Malnutrition and Weight Loss: Persistent inflammation and discomfort caused by gastritis can lead to a decreased appetite, reduced food intake, and malabsorption of nutrients. Over time, this can result in weight loss and nutritional deficiencies.

CHAPTER 3

Meal planning for a gastritis disease diet involves thoughtful selection of foods that are gentle on the stomach, avoid triggers, and promote healing. This proactive approach offers several benefits for the proper management of gastritis:

Benefits of Meal Planning for Gastritis Disease Diet

1. Reduces Irritation: Planning meals ensures the inclusion of foods that are less likely to irritate the stomach lining. This helps in minimizing discomfort and inflammation associated with gastritis.

2. Alleviates Symptoms: Careful selection of foods can help alleviate common symptoms like abdominal pain, bloating, nausea, and indigestion, contributing to improved comfort and quality of life.

3. Supports Digestive Health: Meal planning focuses on easily digestible foods such as lean proteins, cooked vegetables, and whole grains. This supports proper digestion and reduces the workload on the stomach.

4. Balanced Nutrition: Planning meals allows for a well-balanced intake of essential nutrients. It ensures that the diet includes a variety of vitamins, minerals, proteins, and healthy fats necessary for overall health.

5. Avoids Trigger Foods: A planned gastritis diet helps in avoiding trigger foods like spicy, acidic, or high-fat items that can worsen gastritis symptoms.

6. Consistency and Control: Meal planning provides consistency in dietary choices, allowing individuals to maintain control over what they eat. Consistent adherence to a gastritis-friendly diet can lead to better symptom management.

7. Reduces Stress and Anxiety: Knowing in advance what foods are suitable for consumption reduces stress and anxiety related to mealtime decisions. This can positively impact digestion by promoting a relaxed eating experience.

8. Saves Time and Effort: Planning meals in advance saves time and effort spent on making decisions about what to eat, especially during moments of discomfort or when experiencing symptoms.

9. Customized to Individual Needs: Meal planning allows for customization according to individual preferences and sensitivities, ensuring a diet that suits one's specific condition and promotes healing.

Tips for Gastritis Disease Diet Meal Planning

- **Include a Variety of Gentle Foods:** Incorporate fruits, vegetables, lean proteins, whole grains, and healthy fats into meals.
- **Portion Control:** Opt for smaller, frequent meals throughout the day to prevent overloading the stomach.
- **Cooking Methods:** Choose cooking methods like baking, steaming, or boiling rather than frying or grilling to ease digestion.
- **Hydration:** Plan to include sufficient water intake between meals to stay hydrated and aid digestion.
- **Regular Eating Schedule:** Maintain a regular eating schedule to support consistent digestion.

30 DAYS MEAL PLAN

Day 1

- Breakfast: Banana Oatmeal

- Lunch: Quinoa Salad with Grilled Chicken

- Dinner: Baked Herb Chicken with Roasted Vegetables

Day 2

- Breakfast: Greek Yogurt Parfait

- Lunch: Baked Salmon with Steamed Vegetables

- Dinner: Quinoa Stir-Fry with Tofu and Broccoli

Day 3

- Breakfast: Scrambled Tofu with Spinach

- Lunch: Turkey and Vegetable Stir-Fry

- Dinner: Baked Salmon with Steamed Asparagus

Day 4

- Breakfast: Apple Cinnamon Quinoa Bowl

- Lunch: Lentil Soup

- Dinner: Turkey and Vegetable Skillet

Day 5

- Breakfast: Whole Grain Toast with Almond Butter and Berries

- Lunch: Tofu and Vegetable Salad Bowl

- Dinner: Veggie and Lentil Curry

Day 6

- Breakfast: Chia Seed Pudding

- Lunch: Chicken and Vegetable Wrap

- Dinner: Roasted Vegetable Quinoa Bowl

Day 7

- Breakfast: Rice Cake with Avocado and Turkey Slices

- Lunch: Spinach and Tofu Stir-Fry

- Dinner: Grilled Lemon Herb Shrimp with Brown Rice

Day 8

- Breakfast: Berry Smoothie Bowl

- Lunch: Turkey and Quinoa Stuffed Bell Peppers

- Dinner: Veggie and Chickpea Curry

Day 9

- Breakfast: Boiled Egg and Toast

- Lunch: Salmon Salad

- Dinner: Turkey Meatballs with Zucchini Noodles

Day 10

- Breakfast: Cottage Cheese with Fruit

- Lunch: Veggie and Lentil Soup

- Dinner: Vegetable Quiche with Whole Wheat Crust

Day 11

- Breakfast: Pancakes with Blueberry Compote

- Lunch: Tofu and Vegetable Brown Rice Bowl

- Dinner: Baked Lemon Herb Tilapia with Steamed Vegetables

Day 12

- Breakfast: Turkey and Spinach Omelets

- Lunch: Greek Yogurt Chicken Salad

- Dinner: Tofu and Vegetable Skewers with Quinoa

Day 13

- Breakfast: Muesli with Almond Milk and Berries

- Lunch: Veggie and Chickpea Stir-Fry

- Dinner: Chicken and Spinach Stir-Fry with Brown Rice

Day 14

- Breakfast: Peanut Butter and Banana Sandwich

- Lunch: Turkey and Avocado Salad

- Dinner: Veggie and Lentil Stuffed Bell Peppers

Day 15

- Breakfast: Veggie and Cheese Oatmeal

- Lunch: Vegetable and Quinoa Soup

- Dinner: Turkey and Bean Chili

Day 16

- Breakfast: Banana-Oat Energy Bites

- Lunch: Tofu and Vegetable Salad Bowl

- Dinner: Veggie and Lentil Curry

Day 17

- Breakfast: Veggie and Cheese Oatmeal

- Lunch: Tofu and Vegetable Brown Rice Bowl

- Dinner: Baked Lemon Herb Tilapia with Steamed Vegetables

Day 18

- Breakfast: Banana and Spinach Smoothie

- Lunch: Greek Yogurt Chicken Salad

- Dinner: Tofu and Vegetable Skewers with Quinoa

Day 19

- Breakfast: Veggie and Cheese Oatmeal

- Lunch: Veggie and Chickpea Stir-Fry

- Dinner: Chicken and Spinach Stir-Fry with Brown Rice

Day 20

- Breakfast: Banana-Oat Energy Bites

- Lunch: Turkey and Avocado Salad

- Dinner: Veggie and Lentil Stuffed Bell Peppers

Day 21

- Breakfast: Pancakes with Blueberry Compote

- Lunch: Veggie and Quinoa Soup

- Dinner: Turkey and Bean Chili

Day 22

- Breakfast: Chia Seed Pudding

- Lunch: Chicken and Vegetable Wrap

- Dinner: Baked Herb Chicken with Roasted Vegetables

Day 23

- Breakfast: Rice Cake with Avocado and Turkey Slices

- Lunch: Spinach and Tofu Stir-Fry

- Dinner: Quinoa Stir-Fry with Tofu and Broccoli

Day 24

- Breakfast: Berry Smoothie Bowl

- Lunch: Turkey and Vegetable Stir-Fry

- Dinner: Baked Salmon with Steamed Asparagus

Day 25

- Breakfast: Boiled Egg and Toast

- Lunch: Lentil Soup

- Dinner: Turkey and Vegetable Skillet

Day 26

- Breakfast: Cottage Cheese with Fruit

- Lunch: Tofu and Vegetable Salad Bowl

- Dinner: Veggie and Lentil Curry

Day 27

- Breakfast: Pancakes with Blueberry Compote

- Lunch: Tofu and Vegetable Brown Rice Bowl

- Dinner: Veggie and Chickpea Curry

Day 28

- Breakfast: Chia Seed Pudding

- Lunch: Chicken and Vegetable Wrap

- Dinner: Roasted Vegetable Quinoa Bowl

Day 29

- Breakfast: Choose any breakfast option from the provided recipes list.

- Lunch: Select a gastritis-friendly lunch recipe.

- Dinner: Pick a nutritious dinner recipe that suits your preferences.

Day 30

- Breakfast: Opt for another breakfast recipe from your list.

- Lunch: Enjoy a delicious lunch option from the available recipes.

- Dinner: Select a gastritis-friendly dinner recipe to complete your 30-day meal plan.

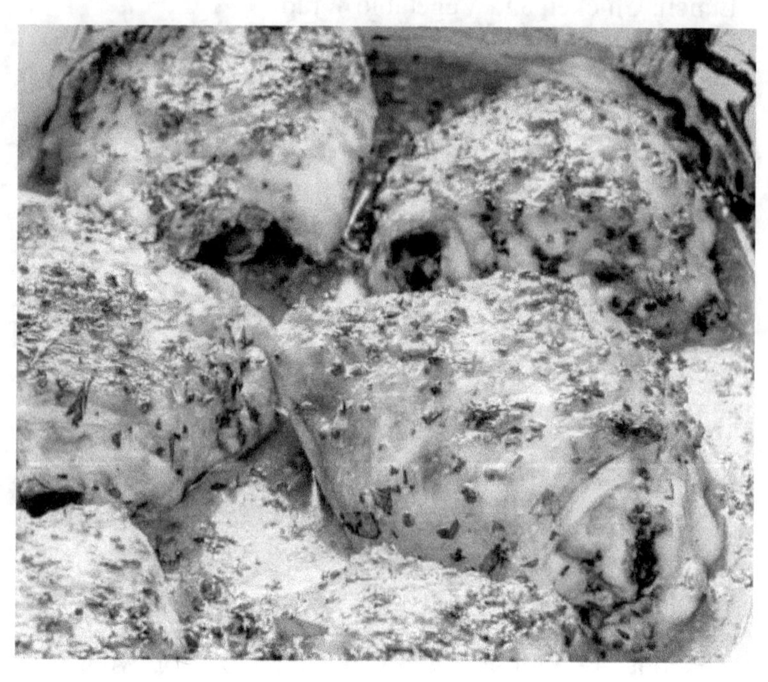

CHAPTER 4

BREAKFAST RECIPES

1. Banana Oatmeal

Ingredients:
- 1 cup rolled oats
- 1 ripe banana, mashed
- 2 cups water or almond milk
- 1 tablespoon honey (optional)
- A sprinkle of cinnamon (optional)
- Sliced almonds or walnuts for topping

Preparation:
1. In a saucepan, combine oats and water/almond milk.
2. Cook over medium heat, stirring occasionally, for 5-7 minutes until the oats are soft and the mixture thickens.
3. Add mashed banana and honey (if using), stirring until well combined.
4. Sprinkle with cinnamon if desired.
5. Serve hot, topped with sliced almonds or walnuts.

Nutritional Value (approx. per serving):
- Calories: 300
- Protein: 7g

- Carbohydrates: 55g
- Fiber: 7g

Cooking Time: 10-12 minutes

2. Greek Yogurt Parfait

Ingredients:
- 1 cup Greek yogurt
- 1/2 cup granola
- 1/2 cup mixed berries (strawberries, blueberries, raspberries)
- 1 tablespoon honey (optional)

Preparation:
1. In a glass or bowl, layer Greek yogurt, granola, and mixed berries.
2. Repeat layers until ingredients are used up.
3. Drizzle honey on top if desired.

Nutritional Value (approx. per serving):
- Calories: 300
- Protein: 20g
- Carbohydrates: 40g
- Fiber: 6g

Preparation Time: 5 minutes

3. Scrambled Tofu with Spinach

Ingredients:
- 1 block firm tofu, crumbled
- 1 cup fresh spinach, chopped
- 1 tablespoon olive oil
- 1/4 teaspoon turmeric powder
- Salt and pepper to taste

Preparation:
1. Heat olive oil in a pan over medium heat.
2. Add crumbled tofu and cook for 3-4 minutes until slightly browned.
3. Add chopped spinach, turmeric powder, salt, and pepper.
4. Cook for another 2-3 minutes until spinach wilts and flavors meld.

Nutritional Value (approx. per serving):
- Calories: 220
- Protein: 18g
- Carbohydrates: 6g
- Fiber: 3g

Cooking Time: 10 minutes

4. Apple Cinnamon Quinoa Bowl

Ingredients:
- 1 cup cooked quinoa
- 1 apple, diced
- 1/4 teaspoon ground cinnamon
- 1 tablespoon honey (optional)
- Sliced almonds for topping

Preparation:
1. In a bowl, combine cooked quinoa, diced apple, cinnamon, and honey (if using).
2. Mix well until ingredients are evenly distributed.
3. Top with sliced almonds.

Nutritional Value (approx. per serving):
- Calories: 280
- Protein: 7g
- Carbohydrates: 50g
- Fiber: 7g

Cooking Time: 15 minutes (if quinoa needs to be cooked)

5. Whole Grain Toast with Almond Butter and Berries

Ingredients:
- 2 slices whole grain bread
- 2 tablespoons almond butter
- Mixed berries (strawberries, blueberries, raspberries) for topping

Preparation:
1. Toast the whole grain bread slices until lightly browned.
2. Spread almond butter evenly on each slice.
3. Top with mixed berries.

Nutritional Value (approx. per serving):
- Calories: 320
- Protein: 11g
- Carbohydrates: 36g
- Fiber: 8g

Cooking Time: 5 minutes

6. Chia Seed Pudding

Ingredients:
- 1/4 cup chia seeds
- 1 cup almond milk (or any preferred milk)
- 1 tablespoon honey or maple syrup
- Fresh fruit (e.g., berries, sliced bananas) for topping

Preparation:
1. In a bowl or jar, mix chia seeds, almond milk, and sweetener.
2. Stir well and let it sit for 15-20 minutes or refrigerate overnight to thicken.
3. Top with fresh fruit before serving.

Nutritional Value (approx. per serving):
- Calories: 180
- Protein: 5g
- Carbohydrates: 25g
- Fiber: 10g

Preparation Time: 5 minutes

7. Rice Cake with Avocado and Turkey Slices

Ingredients:
- 2 rice cakes
- 1/2 ripe avocado, mashed
- 4-6 slices of turkey breast
- Salt and pepper to taste

Preparation:
1. Spread mashed avocado evenly over the rice cakes.
2. Layer turkey slices on top of the avocado.
3. Season with salt and pepper if desired.

Nutritional Value (approx. per serving):
- Calories: 280
- Protein: 15g
- Carbohydrates: 20g
- Fiber: 5g

Preparation Time: 5 minutes

8. Berry Smoothie Bowl

Ingredients:
- 1 cup mixed berries (frozen or fresh)
- 1 ripe banana
- 1/2 cup Greek yogurt
- 1/4 cup almond milk (or any preferred milk)
- Toppings: Granola, sliced almonds, shredded coconut

Preparation:
1. Blend mixed berries, banana, Greek yogurt, and almond milk until smooth.
2. Pour the smoothie into a bowl.
3. Top with granola, sliced almonds, and shredded coconut.

Nutritional Value (approx. per serving):
- Calories: 290
- Protein: 12g
- Carbohydrates: 45g
- Fiber: 9g

Preparation Time: 5 minutes

9. Boiled Egg and Toast

Ingredients:
- 2 hard-boiled eggs
- 2 slices whole grain toast
- Salt and pepper to taste
- Fresh herbs (optional)

Preparation:
1. Peel the hard-boiled eggs and slice them.
2. Toast the whole grain bread slices.
3. Place sliced eggs on top of the toast.
4. Season with salt, pepper, and fresh herbs if desired.

Nutritional Value (approx. per serving):
- Calories: 260
- Protein: 16g
- Carbohydrates: 24g
- Fiber: 4g

Preparation Time: 10 minutes (including boiling eggs)

10. Cottage Cheese with Fruit

Ingredients:
- 1 cup cottage cheese
- Assorted fruits (e.g., sliced peaches, berries, pineapple chunks)
- Honey or maple syrup for drizzling (optional)

Preparation:
1. Place cottage cheese in a bowl.
2. Top with assorted fruits.
3. Drizzle honey or maple syrup if desired.

Nutritional Value (approx. per serving):
- Calories: 220
- Protein: 22g
- Carbohydrates: 20g
- Fiber: 3g

Preparation Time: 5 minutes

11. Pancakes with Blueberry Compote

Ingredients for Pancakes:
- 1 cup oat flour (blend rolled oats to make flour)
- 1 ripe banana, mashed
- 1 teaspoon baking powder
- 1/2 cup almond milk (or any preferred milk)
- 1 tablespoon maple syrup (optional)
- Cooking spray or a little oil for the pan

Ingredients for Blueberry Compote:
- 1 cup fresh or frozen blueberries
- 1 tablespoon honey
- 2 tablespoons water

Preparation:
1. In a bowl, mix oat flour, mashed banana, baking powder, almond milk, and maple syrup (if using) until well combined.
2. Heat a non-stick pan over medium heat and lightly coat it with cooking spray or oil.
3. Pour batter onto the pan to make pancakes. Cook until bubbles form, then flip and cook until golden brown.
4. For the compote, in a saucepan, combine blueberries, honey, and water. Simmer for 5-7 minutes until the mixture thickens.
5. Serve pancakes topped with warm blueberry compote.

Nutritional Value (approx. per serving):
- Calories: 320
- Protein: 7g
- Carbohydrates: 65g
- Fiber: 8g

Preparation Time: 20 minutes

12. Turkey and Spinach Omelets

Ingredients:
- 2 eggs
- 1/4 cup cooked turkey breast, diced
- 1/2 cup fresh spinach, chopped
- Salt and pepper to taste
- 1 teaspoon olive oil

Preparation:
1. In a bowl, whisk the eggs until well beaten. Season with salt and pepper.
2. Heat olive oil in a non-stick pan over medium heat.
3. Add diced turkey breast and chopped spinach, sauté for 1-2 minutes until spinach wilts.
4. Pour beaten eggs into the pan, swirling to cover the bottom evenly.
5. Cook until the edges start to set, then fold the omelet in half. Cook for another minute until fully set.

6. Serve hot.

Nutritional Value (approx. per serving):
- Calories: 250
- Protein: 22g
- Carbohydrates: 2g
- Fiber: 1g

Preparation Time: 10 minutes

13. Muesli with Almond Milk and Berries

Ingredients:
- 1/2 cup muesli
- 1 cup almond milk (or any preferred milk)
- Mixed berries (strawberries, blueberries, raspberries) for topping
- 1 tablespoon honey (optional)

Preparation:
1. In a bowl, combine muesli and almond milk. Let it sit for 5 minutes or overnight in the refrigerator to soften.
2. Top with mixed berries and drizzle honey if desired.

Nutritional Value (approx. per serving):
- Calories: 280

- Protein: 8g
- Carbohydrates: 45g
- Fiber: 6g

Preparation Time: 5 minutes (or overnight soaking)

14. Peanut Butter and Banana Sandwich

Ingredients:
- 2 slices whole grain bread
- 2 tablespoons natural peanut butter
- 1 ripe banana, sliced

Preparation:
1. Toast the whole grain bread slices until golden brown.
2. Spread peanut butter evenly on each slice.
3. Place banana slices on one slice and cover it with the other slice to make a sandwich.

Nutritional Value (approx. per serving):
- Calories: 340
- Protein: 12g
- Carbohydrates: 45g
- Fiber: 8g

Preparation Time: 5 minutes

15. Veggie and Cheese Oatmeal

Ingredients:
- 1/2 cup rolled oats
- 1 cup water or vegetable broth
- 1/4 cup diced mixed vegetables (bell peppers, zucchini, and carrots)
- 2 tablespoons grated cheese (cheddar or mozzarella)
- Salt and pepper to taste

Preparation:
1. In a saucepan, bring water or vegetable broth to a boil.
2. Add rolled oats and diced vegetables. Cook for 5-7 minutes until oats are tender.
3. Stir in grated cheese until melted and well combined.
4. Season with salt and pepper.
5. Serve hot.

Nutritional Value (approx. per serving):
- Calories: 280
- Protein: 10g
- Carbohydrates: 40g
- Fiber: 6g

Preparation Time: 10 minutes

LUNCH RECIPES

1. Quinoa Salad with Grilled Chicken

Ingredients:
- 1 cup cooked quinoa
- 4 oz. grilled chicken breast, diced
- 1/2 cup cucumber, diced
- 1/2 cup cherry tomatoes, halved
- 2 cups mixed greens (spinach, arugula, or lettuce)
- 1 tablespoon olive oil
- 1 tablespoon lemon juice
- Salt and pepper to taste

Preparation:
1. In a large bowl, combine cooked quinoa, grilled chicken, cucumber, cherry tomatoes, and mixed greens.
2. Drizzle olive oil and lemon juice over the salad.
3. Season with salt and pepper.
4. Toss gently until ingredients are well mixed.
5. Serve chilled.

Nutritional Value (approx. per serving):
- Calories: 380
- Protein: 28g
- Carbohydrates: 30g

- Fiber: 5g

Cooking Time: 20 minutes (including quinoa cooking time)

2. Baked Salmon with Steamed Vegetables

Ingredients:
- 6 oz. salmon fillet
- 1 tablespoon olive oil
- 1/2 teaspoon dried herbs (such as dill or thyme)
- 1 cup mixed vegetables (broccoli, carrots, bell peppers)
- Lemon wedges for garnish
- Salt and pepper to taste

Preparation:
1. Preheat oven to 375°F (190°C).
2. Place the salmon fillet on a baking sheet lined with parchment paper.
3. Drizzle olive oil over the salmon and sprinkle with dried herbs, salt, and pepper.
4. Bake for 15-20 minutes until the salmon is cooked through.
5. Meanwhile, steam mixed vegetables until tender-crisp.
6. Serve the baked salmon with steamed vegetables and lemon wedges.

Nutritional Value (approx. per serving):
- Calories: 320
- Protein: 30g
- Carbohydrates: 10g
- Fiber: 3g

Cooking Time: 20 minutes

3. Turkey and Vegetable Stir-Fry

Ingredients:
- 4 oz. cooked turkey breast, sliced
- 1 cup mixed vegetables (bell peppers, broccoli, snap peas)
- 1 tablespoon olive oil
- 2 tablespoons low-sodium soy sauce
- 1 teaspoon honey
- 1/2 teaspoon grated ginger
- Cooked brown rice (optional, for serving)

Preparation:
1. Heat olive oil in a pan over medium-high heat.
2. Add turkey slices and mixed vegetables to the pan. Stir-fry for 4-5 minutes until vegetables are tender.
3. In a small bowl, mix soy sauce, honey, and grated ginger.
4. Pour the sauce over the turkey and vegetables. Stir until everything is coated and heated through.
5. Serve the stir-fry alone or with cooked brown rice.

Nutritional Value (approx. per serving without rice):
- Calories: 250
- Protein: 28g
- Carbohydrates: 10g
- Fiber: 3g

Cooking Time: 15 minutes

4. Lentil Soup

Ingredients:
- 1 cup dried lentils, rinsed
- 4 cups vegetable broth
- 1 onion, chopped
- 2 carrots, diced
- 2 celery stalks, diced
- 2 cloves garlic, minced
- 1 tablespoon olive oil
- 1 teaspoon dried thyme
- Salt and pepper to taste

Preparation:
1. Heat olive oil in a large pot over medium heat.
2. Sauté chopped onion, carrots, celery, and garlic for 5 minutes until softened.
3. Add lentils, vegetable broth, dried thyme, salt, and pepper to the pot.

4. Bring to a boil, then reduce heat and simmer for 25-30 minutes until lentils are tender.
5. Adjust seasoning if needed.
6. Serve hot.

Nutritional Value (approx. per serving):
- Calories: 300
- Protein: 18g
- Carbohydrates: 40g
- Fiber: 15g

Cooking Time: 35 minutes

5. Tofu and Vegetable Salad Bowl

Ingredients:
- 6 oz. firm tofu, cubed
- 2 cups mixed salad greens
- 1/2 cup cucumber, sliced
- 1/2 cup cherry tomatoes, halved
- 2 tablespoons balsamic vinaigrette
- 1 tablespoon chopped fresh basil
- Salt and pepper to taste

Preparation:
1. Season tofu cubes with salt and pepper.
2. Heat a non-stick pan over medium-high heat and lightly coat with cooking spray.

3. Cook tofu cubes for 4-5 minutes, turning occasionally, until golden brown.

4. In a bowl, combine mixed salad greens, cucumber, cherry tomatoes, and cooked tofu.

5. Drizzle with balsamic vinaigrette and sprinkle chopped basil on top.

6. Toss gently until well combined.

7. Serve immediately as a salad bowl or arrange on a plate.

Nutritional Value (approx. per serving):
- Calories: 280
- Protein: 18g
- Carbohydrates: 20g
- Fiber: 6g

Cooking Time: 10 minutes

6. Chicken and Vegetable Wrap

Ingredients:
- 4 oz. cooked chicken breast, shredded
- 2 whole grain tortillas
- 1/2 cup mixed vegetables (bell peppers, lettuce, and carrots)
- 2 tablespoons hummus or avocado spread

Preparation:
1. Lay out the whole grain tortillas.
2. Spread hummus or avocado spread evenly on each tortilla.
3. Add shredded chicken and mixed vegetables.
4. Roll up tightly into wraps and cut in half.

Nutritional Value (approx. per serving):
- Calories: 320
- Protein: 25g
- Carbohydrates: 30g
- Fiber: 6g

Cooking Time: 10 minutes

7. Spinach and Tofu Stir-Fry

Ingredients:
- 6 oz. firm tofu, cubed
- 2 cups fresh spinach
- 1/2 cup sliced mushrooms
- 1/4 cup sliced bell peppers
- 1 tablespoon olive oil
- 2 tablespoons low-sodium soy sauce
- 1 clove garlic, minced
- 1/2 teaspoon grated ginger

Preparation:
1. Heat olive oil in a pan over medium-high heat.
2. Add minced garlic and grated ginger, stir for 30 seconds.
3. Add tofu cubes and stir-fry until lightly browned.
4. Add sliced mushrooms and bell peppers, cook for 2-3 minutes.
5. Toss in fresh spinach until wilted.
6. Drizzle with soy sauce, stir to combine, and cook for another minute.
7. Serve hot.

Nutritional Value (approx. per serving):
- Calories: 270
- Protein: 20g
- Carbohydrates: 12g
- Fiber: 4g

Cooking Time: 20 minutes

8. Turkey and Quinoa Stuffed Bell Peppers

Ingredients:
- 2 bell peppers, halved and seeds removed
- 1/2 cup cooked quinoa
- 4 oz. cooked turkey breast, diced
- 1/4 cup diced tomatoes
- 2 tablespoons chopped parsley
- Salt and pepper to taste
- 2 tablespoons grated mozzarella cheese (optional)

Preparation:
1. Preheat oven to 375°F (190°C).
2. In a bowl, mix cooked quinoa, diced turkey, diced tomatoes, chopped parsley, salt, and pepper.
3. Stuff the halved bell peppers with the quinoa and turkey mixture.
4. Place the stuffed peppers on a baking dish and bake for 25-30 minutes until peppers are tender.
5. Optionally, sprinkle grated mozzarella cheese on top before baking for added flavor.

Nutritional Value (approx. per serving):
- Calories: 290

- Protein: 25g
- Carbohydrates: 30g
- Fiber: 6g

Cooking Time: 35 minutes

9. Salmon Salad

Ingredients:
- 4 oz. canned salmon, drained
- 2 cups mixed salad greens
- 1/4 cup cucumber, sliced
- 1/4 cup cherry tomatoes, halved
- 1 tablespoon olive oil
- 1 tablespoon lemon juice
- Salt and pepper to taste

Preparation:
1. In a bowl, combine mixed salad greens, sliced cucumber, cherry tomatoes, and canned salmon.
2. Drizzle with olive oil and lemon juice.
3. Season with salt and pepper.
4. Toss gently until well mixed.
5. Serve immediately.

Nutritional Value (approx. per serving):
- Calories: 270
- Protein: 25g

- Carbohydrates: 8g
- Fiber: 3g

Cooking Time: 15 minutes

10. Veggie and Lentil Soup

Ingredients:
- 1 cup cooked lentils
- 4 cups vegetable broth
- 1 onion, chopped
- 2 carrots, diced
- 2 celery stalks, diced
- 1 cup diced tomatoes
- 2 cloves garlic, minced
- 1 tablespoon olive oil
- 1 teaspoon dried herbs (such as thyme or oregano)
- Salt and pepper to taste

Preparation:
1. Heat olive oil in a pot over medium heat.
2. Sauté chopped onion, carrots, celery, and minced garlic for 5 minutes.
3. Add diced tomatoes, cooked lentils, vegetable broth, dried herbs, salt, and pepper to the pot.
4. Bring to a boil, then reduce heat and simmer for 20-25 minutes.
5. Adjust seasoning if needed.

6. Serve hot.

Nutritional Value (approx. per serving):
- Calories: 280
- Protein: 18g
- Carbohydrates: 45g
- Fiber: 14g

Cooking Time: 30 minutes

11. Tofu and Vegetable Brown Rice Bowl

Ingredients:
- 6 oz. firm tofu, cubed
- 1 cup cooked brown rice
- 1/2 cup mixed vegetables (broccoli, carrots, bell peppers)
- 1 tablespoon low-sodium soy sauce
- 1 tablespoon sesame oil
- 1 teaspoon grated ginger
- 1 clove garlic, minced

Preparation:
1. Heat sesame oil in a pan over medium-high heat.
2. Add minced garlic and grated ginger, stir for 30 seconds.
3. Add tofu cubes and stir-fry until golden brown.

4. Add mixed vegetables and continue stir-frying for 2-3 minutes.
5. Add cooked brown rice and soy sauce, mix well until heated through.
6. Serve hot.

Nutritional Value (approx. per serving):
- Calories: 320
- Protein: 18g
- Carbohydrates: 40g
- Fiber: 5g

Cooking Time: 20 minutes

12. Greek Yogurt Chicken Salad

Ingredients:
- 4 oz. cooked chicken breast, shredded
- 1/2 cup Greek yogurt
- 1/4 cup diced cucumber
- 1/4 cup diced red onion
- 1 tablespoon chopped fresh dill
- Salt and pepper to taste

Preparation:
1. In a bowl, mix shredded chicken, Greek yogurt, diced cucumber, diced red onion, and chopped fresh dill.
2. Season with salt and pepper.

3. Serve as a salad or in a whole grain pita pocket.

Nutritional Value (approx. per serving):
- Calories: 280
- Protein: 30g
- Carbohydrates: 10g
- Fiber: 1g

Preparation Time: 30 minutes

13. Veggie and Chickpea Stir-Fry

Ingredients:
- 1 can (15 oz.) chickpeas, drained and rinsed
- 1 cup mixed vegetables (bell peppers, broccoli, snap peas)
- 1 tablespoon olive oil
- 2 tablespoons low-sodium soy sauce
- 1 teaspoon honey
- 1/2 teaspoon grated ginger
- 1 clove garlic, minced

Preparation:
1. Heat olive oil in a pan over medium-high heat.
2. Add minced garlic and grated ginger, stir for 30 seconds.
3. Add mixed vegetables and chickpeas, stir-fry for 3-4 minutes.
4. In a small bowl, mix soy sauce and honey.

5. Pour the sauce over the vegetables and chickpeas, toss to coat.
6. Cook for an additional minute until heated through.
7. Serve hot.

Nutritional Value (approx. per serving):
- Calories: 290
- Protein: 12g
- Carbohydrates: 40g
- Fiber: 10g

Cooking Time: 20 minutes

14. Turkey and Avocado Salad

Ingredients:
- 4 oz. cooked turkey breast, sliced
- 2 cups mixed salad greens
- 1/2 avocado, sliced
- 1/4 cup cherry tomatoes, halved
- 1 tablespoon balsamic vinaigrette
- Salt and pepper to taste

Preparation:
1. Arrange mixed salad greens on a plate.
2. Top with sliced turkey, avocado, and cherry tomatoes.
3. Drizzle with balsamic vinaigrette.
4. Season with salt and pepper.

5. Serve immediately.

Nutritional Value (approx. per serving):
- Calories: 290
- Protein: 25g
- Carbohydrates: 12g
- Fiber: 6g

Cooking Time: 20 minutes

15. Vegetable and Quinoa Soup

Ingredients:
- 1 cup cooked quinoa
- 4 cups vegetable broth
- 1 onion, chopped
- 2 carrots, diced
- 2 celery stalks, diced
- 1 cup diced tomatoes
- 1 cup chopped spinach
- 2 cloves garlic, minced
- 1 tablespoon olive oil
- 1 teaspoon dried herbs (such as basil or oregano)
- Salt and pepper to taste

Preparation:
1. Heat olive oil in a pot over medium heat.

2. Sauté chopped onion, carrots, celery, and minced garlic for 5 minutes.

3. Add diced tomatoes, chopped spinach, cooked quinoa, vegetable broth, dried herbs, salt, and pepper to the pot.

4. Bring to a boil, then reduce heat and simmer for 20-25 minutes.

5. Adjust seasoning if needed.

6. Serve hot.

Nutritional Value (approx. per serving):
- Calories: 270
- Protein: 10g
- Carbohydrates: 40g
- Fiber: 8g

Cooking Time: 30 minutes

DINNER RECIPES

1. Baked Herb Chicken with Roasted Vegetables

Ingredients:
- 2 boneless, skinless chicken breasts
- 2 cups mixed vegetables (zucchini, bell peppers, carrots)
- 1 tablespoon olive oil
- 1 teaspoon dried herbs (thyme, rosemary)
- Salt and pepper to taste

Preparation:
1. Preheat oven to 375°F (190°C).
2. Place chicken breasts on a baking sheet lined with parchment paper.
3. Toss mixed vegetables with olive oil, dried herbs, salt, and pepper.
4. Spread vegetables around the chicken on the baking sheet.
5. Bake for 25-30 minutes until the chicken is cooked through and vegetables are tender.

Nutritional Value (approx. per serving):
- Calories: 280
- Protein: 30g
- Carbohydrates: 15g
- Fiber: 5g

Cooking Time: 30 minutes

2. Quinoa Stir-Fry with Tofu and Broccoli

Ingredients:
- 1 cup cooked quinoa
- 6 oz. firm tofu, cubed
- 2 cups broccoli florets
- 2 tablespoons low-sodium soy sauce
- 1 tablespoon sesame oil
- 1 clove garlic, minced
- 1 teaspoon grated ginger
- 1 tablespoon chopped green onions (optional)

Preparation:
1. Heat sesame oil in a pan over medium-high heat.
2. Add minced garlic and grated ginger, stir for 30 seconds.
3. Add cubed tofu and stir-fry until golden brown.
4. Add broccoli florets and cooked quinoa, continue stir-frying for 3-4 minutes.
5. Pour low-sodium soy sauce over the mixture and toss to combine.
6. Cook for an additional 2 minutes.
7. Garnish with chopped green onions if desired.

Nutritional Value (approx. per serving):

- Calories: 320
- Protein: 22g
- Carbohydrates: 30g
- Fiber: 6g

Cooking Time: 20 minutes

3. Baked Salmon with Steamed Asparagus

Ingredients:
- 2 salmon fillets
- 1 tablespoon olive oil
- 1 lemon, sliced
- Salt and pepper to taste
- 1 bunch asparagus

Preparation:
1. Preheat oven to 400°F (200°C).
2. Place salmon fillets on a baking sheet lined with parchment paper.
3. Drizzle olive oil over the salmon and season with salt and pepper.
4. Place lemon slices on top of each fillet.
5. Bake for 12-15 minutes until salmon is cooked through.
6. Steam asparagus until tender-crisp.

7. Serve baked salmon with steamed asparagus.

Nutritional Value (approx. per serving):
- Calories: 300
- Protein: 30g
- Carbohydrates: 8g
- Fiber: 4g

Cooking Time: 15 minutes

4. Turkey and Vegetable Skillet

Ingredients:
- 8 oz. ground turkey
- 1 cup mixed vegetables (bell peppers, carrots, peas)
- 1/2 onion, chopped
- 1 clove garlic, minced
- 1 tablespoon olive oil
- 2 tablespoons tomato paste
- 1/4 cup low-sodium chicken broth
- Salt and pepper to taste

Preparation:
1. Heat olive oil in a skillet over medium-high heat.
2. Add chopped onion and minced garlic, sauté for 2 minutes.
3. Add ground turkey and cook until browned.
4. Stir in mixed vegetables, tomato paste, and chicken broth.

5. Cook for 5-7 minutes until vegetables are tender.

6. Season with salt and pepper.

7. Serve hot.

Nutritional Value (approx. per serving):

- Calories: 260

- Protein: 25g

- Carbohydrates: 12g

- Fiber: 3g

Cooking Time: 20 minutes

5. Veggie and Lentil Curry

Ingredients:

- 1 cup cooked lentils

- 1 cup mixed vegetables (bell peppers, cauliflower, peas)

- 1/2 onion, chopped

- 1 clove garlic, minced

- 1 tablespoon olive oil

- 2 tablespoons curry paste

- 1 cup coconut milk

- Salt and pepper to taste

Preparation:

1. Heat olive oil in a pan over medium heat.

2. Sauté chopped onion and minced garlic until softened.

3. Add mixed vegetables and cook for 5 minutes.

4. Stir in curry paste and cook for another minute.

5. Add cooked lentils and coconut milk, stirring to combine.

6. Simmer for 10-15 minutes until vegetables are tender and flavors meld.

7. Season with salt and pepper.

8. Serve with rice or quinoa if desired.

Nutritional Value (approx. per serving):
- Calories: 320
- Protein: 15g
- Carbohydrates: 25g
- Fiber: 8g

Cooking Time: 25 minutes

6. Roasted Vegetable Quinoa Bowl

Ingredients:
- 1 cup cooked quinoa
- 2 cups assorted vegetables (bell peppers, zucchini, and cherry tomatoes)
- 1 tablespoon olive oil
- 1 teaspoon dried herbs (oregano, basil)
- Salt and pepper to taste
- Optional: 2 tablespoons crumbled feta cheese

Preparation:
1. Preheat oven to 400°F (200°C).

2. Toss assorted vegetables with olive oil, dried herbs, salt, and pepper.

3. Spread vegetables on a baking sheet lined with parchment paper.

4. Roast for 20-25 minutes until vegetables are tender and slightly browned.

5. Divide cooked quinoa into bowls, top with roasted vegetables.

6. Optionally, sprinkle with crumbled feta cheese before serving.

Nutritional Value (approx. per serving):
- Calories: 290
- Protein: 8g
- Carbohydrates: 45g
- Fiber: 8g
- Cooking Time: 25 minutes

7. Grilled Lemon Herb Shrimp with Brown Rice

Ingredients:
- 8 oz.. shrimp, peeled and deveined
- 1 tablespoon olive oil
- 1 lemon (juice and zest)
- 1 teaspoon dried herbs (thyme, rosemary)
- 2 cups cooked brown rice
- Salt and pepper to taste

Preparation:
1. In a bowl, combine shrimp, olive oil, lemon zest, lemon juice, dried herbs, salt, and pepper.
2. Preheat grill or grill pan over medium-high heat.
3. Thread shrimp onto skewers and grill for 2-3 minutes on each side until cooked.
4. Serve grilled shrimp over cooked brown rice.

Nutritional Value (approx. per serving):
- Calories: 320
- Protein: 25g
- Carbohydrates: 30g
- Fiber: 3g

Cooking Time: 10 minutes

8. Veggie and Chickpea Curry

Ingredients:
- 1 can (15 oz..) chickpeas, drained and rinsed
- 2 cups mixed vegetables (cauliflower, bell peppers, peas)
- 1/2 onion, chopped
- 2 cloves garlic, minced
- 1 tablespoon olive oil
- 2 tablespoons curry powder
- 1 cup vegetable broth
- 1/2 cup coconut milk
- Salt and pepper to taste

Preparation:
1. Heat olive oil in a pan over medium heat.
2. Sauté chopped onion and minced garlic until softened.
3. Add mixed vegetables and chickpeas, cook for 5 minutes.
4. Stir in curry powder, vegetable broth, and coconut milk.
5. Simmer for 15-20 minutes until vegetables are tender and sauce thickens.
6. Season with salt and pepper.
7. Serve over rice or quinoa if desired.

Nutritional Value (approx. per serving):
- Calories: 280
- Protein: 10g
- Carbohydrates: 35g
- Fiber: 9g

Cooking Time: 25 minutes

9. Turkey Meatballs with Zucchini Noodles

Ingredients:
- 8 oz.. ground turkey
- 1/4 cup breadcrumbs
- 1 egg
- 1/4 cup grated Parmesan cheese
- 2 cups zucchini noodles
- 1 cup marinara sauce
- 1 tablespoon olive oil
- Salt and pepper to taste

Preparation:
1. In a bowl, combine ground turkey, breadcrumbs, egg, grated Parmesan, salt, and pepper. Form into meatballs.
2. Heat olive oil in a skillet over medium heat.
3. Cook meatballs for 10-12 minutes until browned and cooked through.
4. In the same skillet, add zucchini noodles and marinara sauce. Cook for 2-3 minutes until heated.
5. Serve turkey meatballs over zucchini noodles.

Nutritional Value (approx. per serving):
- Calories: 320

- Protein: 25g
- Carbohydrates: 15g
- Fiber: 4g

Cooking Time: 15 minutes

10. Vegetable Quiche with Whole Wheat Crust

Ingredients:
- 1 whole wheat pie crust (store-bought or homemade)
- 1 cup mixed vegetables (bell peppers, spinach, tomatoes)
- 4 eggs
- 1/2 cup milk (or non-dairy alternative)
- 1/4 cup grated cheese (cheddar or Swiss)
- Salt and pepper to taste

Preparation:
1. Preheat oven to 375°F (190°C).
2. Place mixed vegetables in the pie crust.
3. In a bowl, whisk together eggs, milk, grated cheese, salt, and pepper.
4. Pour the egg mixture over the vegetables in the pie crust.
5. Bake for 30-35 minutes until the quiche is set and golden brown.
6. Allow it to cool for a few minutes before slicing.

Nutritional Value (approx. per serving):
- Calories: 280
- Protein: 12g
- Carbohydrates: 20g
- Fiber: 3g

Cooking Time: 35 minutes

11. Baked Lemon Herb Tilapia with Steamed Vegetables

Ingredients:
- 2 tilapia fillets
- 1 tablespoon olive oil
- 1 lemon (juice and zest)
- 1 teaspoon dried herbs (such as parsley or dill)
- Salt and pepper to taste
- 2 cups mixed steamed vegetables (broccoli, carrots, and cauliflower)

Preparation:
1. Preheat oven to 375°F (190°C).
2. Place tilapia fillets on a baking sheet lined with parchment paper.
3. Drizzle olive oil over the fillets and sprinkle with dried herbs, salt, and pepper.

4. Squeeze lemon juice over the fish and sprinkle lemon zest on top.

5. Bake for 12-15 minutes until fish is cooked through.

6. Serve baked tilapia with a side of steamed mixed vegetables.

Nutritional Value (approx. per serving):
- Calories: 250
- Protein: 25g
- Carbohydrates: 8g
- Fiber: 4g

Cooking Time: 15 minutes

12. Tofu and Vegetable Skewers with Quinoa

Ingredients:
- 6 oz.. firm tofu, cubed
- 1 cup mixed vegetables (mushrooms, bell peppers, onions)
- 1 tablespoon olive oil
- 2 cups cooked quinoa
- 2 tablespoons low-sodium soy sauce
- 1 teaspoon honey
- 1/2 teaspoon grated ginger

Preparation:
1. Preheat grill or grill pan over medium-high heat.
2. Thread tofu cubes and mixed vegetables onto skewers.
3. Mix olive oil, soy sauce, honey, and grated ginger in a bowl.
4. Brush skewers with the sauce mixture and grill for 8-10 minutes, turning occasionally.
5. Serve grilled tofu and vegetable skewers over cooked quinoa.

Nutritional Value (approx. per serving):
- Calories: 320
- Protein: 18g
- Carbohydrates: 35g
- Fiber: 6g

Cooking Time: 15 minutes

13. Chicken and Spinach Stir-Fry with Brown Rice

Ingredients:
- 8 oz.. chicken breast, sliced
- 2 cups fresh spinach
- 1/2 cup sliced mushrooms
- 1/4 cup sliced bell peppers
- 1 tablespoon olive oil
- 2 tablespoons low-sodium soy sauce
- 1 teaspoon honey
- 1 clove garlic, minced

Preparation:
1. Heat olive oil in a pan over medium-high heat.
2. Add minced garlic and sliced chicken, stir-fry until chicken is cooked.
3. Add sliced mushrooms and bell peppers, cook for 2-3 minutes.
4. Toss in fresh spinach until wilted.
5. In a small bowl, mix soy sauce and honey.
6. Pour the sauce over the chicken and vegetables, stir to combine.
7. Cook for an additional minute.
8. Serve over cooked brown rice.

Nutritional Value (approx. per serving):
- Calories: 300

- Protein: 25g
- Carbohydrates: 30g
- Fiber: 4g

Cooking Time: 20 minutes

14. Veggie and Lentil Stuffed Bell Peppers

Ingredients:
- 4 bell peppers, halved and seeds removed
- 1 cup cooked lentils
- 1 cup mixed vegetables (tomatoes, onions, carrots)
- 1/2 cup grated mozzarella cheese
- 1 tablespoon olive oil
- Salt and pepper to taste

Preparation:
1. Preheat oven to 375°F (190°C).
2. In a bowl, mix cooked lentils, mixed vegetables, olive oil, salt, and pepper.
3. Stuff each bell pepper half with the lentil and vegetable mixture.
4. Place stuffed bell peppers in a baking dish and cover with foil.
5. Bake for 25-30 minutes until peppers are tender.

6. Remove foil, sprinkle grated mozzarella cheese on top, and bake for an additional 5 minutes until cheese is melted.

Nutritional Value (approx. per serving):
- Calories: 280
- Protein: 15g
- Carbohydrates: 35g
- Fiber: 10g

Cooking Time: 35 minutes

15. Turkey and Bean Chili

Ingredients:
- 1 lb. ground turkey
- 1 can (15 oz.) kidney beans, drained and rinsed
- 1 can (15 oz.) diced tomatoes
- 1 onion, chopped
- 2 cloves garlic, minced
- 2 tablespoons chili powder
- 1 teaspoon cumin
- Salt and pepper to taste

Preparation:
1. In a pot, cook chopped onion and minced garlic until softened.

2. Add ground turkey and cook until browned.
3. Stir in chili powder, cumin, salt, and pepper.
4. Add diced tomatoes and kidney beans.
5. Simmer for 20-25 minutes, stirring occasionally.
6. Adjust seasoning if needed.
7. Serve hot.

Nutritional Value (approx. per serving):
- Calories: 290
- Protein: 25g
- Carbohydrates: 20g
- Fiber: 8g

Cooking Time: 30 minutes

SNACKS RECIPES

1. Rice Cake with Avocado and Turkey

Ingredients:
- 1 rice cake
- 1/4 ripe avocado, mashed
- 2 oz. sliced turkey breast
- Pinch of salt and pepper

Preparation:
1. Spread mashed avocado on the rice cake.
2. Place sliced turkey on top of the avocado.
3. Season with a pinch of salt and pepper.
4. Enjoy immediately.

Nutritional Value (approx. per serving):
- Calories: 150
- Protein: 12g
- Carbohydrates: 10g
- Fiber: 3g

Preparation Time: 15 minutes

2. Banana-Oat Energy Bites

Ingredients:
- 1 ripe banana, mashed
- 1 cup rolled oats
- 2 tablespoons almond butter or peanut butter
- 1 tablespoon honey
- 1/4 cup chopped nuts (walnuts, almonds)

Preparation:
1. In a bowl, mix mashed banana, rolled oats, almond butter, honey, and chopped nuts until well combined.
2. Roll the mixture into bite-sized balls using your hands.
3. Place the energy bites on a baking sheet lined with parchment paper.
4. Refrigerate for at least 30 minutes before serving.

Nutritional Value (approx. per serving - 2 bites):
- Calories: 120
- Protein: 4g
- Carbohydrates: 15g
- Fiber: 2g

Preparation Time: 15 minutes

3. Cottage Cheese and Apple Slices

Ingredients:
- 1/2 cup low-fat cottage cheese
- 1 medium apple, sliced

Preparation:
1. Place cottage cheese in a bowl.
2. Slice the apple and serve it with the cottage cheese.
3. Enjoy this simple and quick snack.

Nutritional Value (approx. per serving):
- Calories: 150
- Protein: 12g
- Carbohydrates: 20g
- Fiber: 4g

Preparation Time: 7 minutes

4. Carrot Sticks with Hummus

Ingredients:
- 2 medium carrots, cut into sticks
- 1/4 cup hummus

Preparation:
1. Wash and cut carrots into sticks.

2. Serve carrot sticks with hummus for dipping.
3. Enjoy this crunchy and healthy snack.

Nutritional Value (approx. per serving):
- Calories: 100
- Protein: 4g
- Carbohydrates: 12g
- Fiber: 4g

Preparation Time: 10 minutes

5. Almond Butter and Banana Rice Cakes

Ingredients:
- 2 rice cakes
- 2 tablespoons almond butter
- 1 ripe banana, sliced
- Cinnamon (optional)

Preparation:
1. Spread almond butter evenly on each rice cake.
2. Top the almond butter with banana slices.
3. Sprinkle a dash of cinnamon for added flavor if desired.
4. Enjoy these tasty and satisfying rice cakes.

Nutritional Value (approx. per serving - 2 rice cakes):

- Calories: 250
- Protein: 6g
- Carbohydrates: 30g
- Fiber: 4g

Preparation Time: 15 minutes

6. Roasted Chickpeas

Ingredients:
- 1 can (15 oz..) chickpeas, drained and rinsed
- 1 tablespoon olive oil
- 1 teaspoon paprika
- 1/2 teaspoon cumin
- Salt to taste

Preparation:
1. Preheat oven to 400°F (200°C).
2. Pat dry the chickpeas using a paper towel.
3. In a bowl, toss chickpeas with olive oil, paprika, cumin, and salt until coated.
4. Spread chickpeas on a baking sheet lined with parchment paper.
5. Roast for 25-30 minutes until crispy, shaking the pan occasionally.
6. Let cool before enjoying these crunchy roasted chickpeas.

Nutritional Value (approx. per serving - 1/2 cup):

- Calories: 150
- Protein: 6g
- Carbohydrates: 20g
- Fiber: 6g

Preparation Time: 15 minutes

DESSERTS AND TREATS RECIPES

1. Banana-Oat Cookies

Ingredients:
- 2 ripe bananas, mashed
- 1 cup rolled oats
- 1/4 cup chopped nuts (walnuts, almonds)
- 1/4 cup unsweetened shredded coconut
- Cinnamon or vanilla extract (optional)

Preparation:
1. Preheat oven to 350°F (175°C) and line a baking sheet with parchment paper.
2. In a bowl, combine mashed bananas, rolled oats, chopped nuts, shredded coconut, and a dash of cinnamon or a splash of vanilla extract if desired.

3. Drop spoonfuls of the mixture onto the prepared baking sheet.

4. Flatten each cookie slightly with a fork.

5. Bake for 15-18 minutes until golden brown.

6. Let cool before serving.

Nutritional Value (approx. per serving - 2 cookies):
- Calories: 160
- Protein: 4g
- Carbohydrates: 20g
- Fiber: 4g

Cooking Time: 20 minutes

2. Baked Apple with Cinnamon

Ingredients:
- 2 apples (Granny Smith or Honey crisp)
- 2 teaspoons honey
- 1 teaspoon cinnamon
- 2 tablespoons chopped nuts (optional)

Preparation:
1. Preheat oven to 375°F (190°C).

2. Core the apples and place them in a baking dish.

3. Drizzle 1 teaspoon of honey over each apple.

4. Sprinkle cinnamon evenly over the apples.

5. Add chopped nuts on top if desired.

6. Bake for 20-25 minutes until apples are tender.
7. Serve warm.

Nutritional Value (approx. per serving - 1 apple):
- Calories: 120
- Protein: 1g
- Carbohydrates: 30g
- Fiber: 6g

Cooking Time: 25 minutes.

3. Yogurt and Berry Parfait

Ingredients:
- 1 cup Greek yogurt
- 1/2 cup mixed berries (strawberries, blueberries)
- 2 tablespoons granola (optional)

Preparation:
1. In a glass or bowl, layer Greek yogurt and mixed berries.
2. Add a layer of granola if desired.
3. Repeat layers until the glass or bowl is filled.
4. Serve immediately.

Nutritional Value (approx. per serving):
- Calories: 200
- Protein: 15g
- Carbohydrates: 25g

- Fiber: 4g

4. Frozen Banana Bites

Ingredients:
- 2 bananas, peeled and cut into slices
- 1/4 cup dark chocolate chips
- 1 tablespoon coconut oil
- Chopped nuts or shredded coconut (optional)

Preparation:
1. Place banana slices on a parchment-lined baking sheet and freeze for 1-2 hours.
2. In a microwave-safe bowl, melt dark chocolate chips and coconut oil together in 30-second intervals until smooth.
3. Dip each froz.en banana slice halfway into the melted chocolate.
4. Place back on the parchment paper and sprinkle with chopped nuts or shredded coconut if desired.
5. Freeze for an additional 30 minutes until chocolate sets.
6. Serve chilled.

Nutritional Value (approx. per serving - 4 bites):
- Calories: 160
- Protein: 2g
- Carbohydrates: 25g
- Fiber: 4g

Cooking Time: 10 minutes (plus freezing time)

5. Mango and Coconut Chia Popsicles

Ingredients:
- 1 ripe mango, peeled and diced
- 1 can (13.5 oz..) coconut milk
- 1/4 cup chia seeds
- 2 tablespoons honey or maple syrup (optional)

Preparation:
1. Blend diced mango until smooth and set aside.
2. In a bowl, mix coconut milk, chia seeds, and honey or maple syrup (if using).
3. Allow the chia seed mixture to sit for 10 minutes until it thickens.
4. In Popsicle molds, layer the mango puree and chia seed mixture.
5. Insert Popsicle sticks and freeze for at least 4-6 hours until solid.
6. Remove from molds and enjoy these refreshing popsicles.

Nutritional Value (approx. per serving - 1 Popsicle):
- Calories: 120
- Protein: 2g

- Carbohydrates: 15g
- Fiber: 4g

Freezing Time: 4-6 hours

6. Baked Cinnamon Apple Chips

Ingredients:
- 2 apples (Granny Smith or Honey crisp)
- 1 teaspoon ground cinnamon
- 1 tablespoon granulated sugar (optional)

Preparation:
1. Preheat oven to 200°F (95°C) and line baking sheets with parchment paper.
2. Wash and thinly slice the apples crosswise, removing seeds.
3. In a bowl, toss apple slices with ground cinnamon and granulated sugar if desired.
4. Place the apple slices in a single layer on the baking sheets.
5. Bake for 1.5 to 2 hours until the apples are dried and slightly crisp.
6. Let them cool completely before enjoying these crispy apple chips.

Nutritional Value (approx. per serving - 1 apple):
- Calories: 50

- Protein: 0g
- Carbohydrates: 15g
- Fiber: 3g

Baking Time: 1.5-2 hours

BEVERAGES AND DRINKS RECIPES

1. Ginger Turmeric Tea

Ingredients:
- 2 cups water
- 1-inch fresh ginger, sliced
- 1 teaspoon ground turmeric or 1-inch fresh turmeric, sliced
- 1 tablespoon honey (optional)
- Juice of half a lemon (optional)

Preparation:
1. In a saucepan, bring water to a boil.
2. Add sliced ginger and turmeric to the boiling water.
3. Reduce heat and let it simmer for 10-15 minutes.
4. Strain the tea into a cup.
5. Add honey or lemon juice if desired.
6. Enjoy this soothing tea.

Nutritional Value (approx. per serving - 1 cup):
- Calories: 10
- Carbohydrates: 2g
- Fat: 0g

Cooking Time: 15 minutes

2. Cucumber Mint Infused Water

Ingredients:
- 1/2 cucumber, thinly sliced
- Handful of fresh mint leaves
- 4 cups water
- Ice cubes (optional)

Preparation:
1. In a pitcher, combine cucumber slices and fresh mint leaves.
2. Add water and stir well.
3. Refrigerate for at least 2 hours or overnight to infuse flavors.
4. Serve over ice if desired.

Nutritional Value (approx. per serving - 1 cup):
- Calories: 0
- Carbohydrates: 0g
- Fat: 0g

Infusion Time: 2 hours minimum

3. Banana and Spinach Smoothie

Ingredients:
- 1 ripe banana
- Handful of spinach leaves
- 1 cup almond milk (or any preferred milk)
- 1 tablespoon honey or maple syrup (optional)
- Ice cubes (optional)

Preparation:
1. In a blender, combine banana, spinach, almond milk, and honey or maple syrup.
2. Blend until smooth and creamy.
3. Add ice cubes if a colder drink is desired.
4. Pour into a glass and enjoy this nutritious smoothie.

Nutritional Value (approx. per serving - 1 cup):
- Calories: 90
- Protein: 2g
- Carbohydrates: 20g
- Fiber: 3g

Preparation Time: 5 minutes

4. Chamomile Tea with Honey

Ingredients:
- 2 cups water
- 2 chamomile tea bags
- 1 tablespoon honey
- Lemon slices (optional)

Preparation:
1. Heat water in a kettle or saucepan until boiling.
2. Place chamomile tea bags in a teapot or heatproof container.
3. Pour boiling water over the tea bags and steep for 5 minutes.
4. Remove the tea bags and add honey to the tea.
5. Stir well until honey is dissolved.
6. Optionally, add lemon slices for extra flavor.
7. Serve and enjoy this calming beverage.

Nutritional Value (approx. per serving - 1 cup):
- Calories: 30
- Carbohydrates: 8g
- Fat: 0g

Brewing Time: 5 minutes

5. Watermelon and Basil Infused Water

Ingredients:
- 2 cups cubed watermelon
- Handful of fresh basil leaves
- 4 cups water
- Ice cubes (optional)

Preparation:
1. In a pitcher, combine cubed watermelon and fresh basil leaves.
2. Add water and stir gently.
3. Allow it to infuse in the refrigerator for at least 1-2 hours.
4. Serve over ice if desired.

Nutritional Value (approx. per serving - 1 cup):
- Calories: 10
- Carbohydrates: 2g
- Fat: 0g

Infusion Time: 1-2 hours

CONCLUSION

In conclusion, this Gastritis Healing Cookbook for Beginners offers a wealth of gastritis-friendly recipes designed to support digestive health while satisfying taste buds. Throughout these recipes, the focus has been on selecting ingredients and cooking methods that are gentle on the stomach, providing nutrient-rich meals that are both flavorful and supportive of the healing process.

From nourishing breakfast options to satisfying lunch and dinner recipes, along with wholesome snacks and delectable desserts, this cookbook has aimed to provide a diverse array of gastritis-friendly choices. Emphasizing ingredients like lean proteins, whole grains, fruits, vegetables, and healthy fats, each recipe has been crafted to promote a balanced diet that aids in soothing gastric inflammation and discomfort.

By incorporating these recipes into your daily routine, you're not just adopting a diet; you're embracing a lifestyle that prioritizes your well-being. The journey to managing gastritis involves more than just what's on your plate—it's about making mindful choices, listening to your body, and nurturing it with foods that promote healing.

Remember, adopting this gastritis healing diet isn't just a step towards alleviating discomfort; it's a commitment to your health and vitality. Your journey towards better digestive health starts with these recipes, but it's sustained by your determination to prioritize your well-being.

So, whether you're newly diagnosed or seeking ways to manage gastritis symptoms, this cookbook serves as a valuable resource to help you embark on a culinary journey that nurtures your stomach and supports overall health. Take charge of your health, savor the flavors, and embrace this gastritis healing diet as a path to a happier and healthier you. You deserve a life filled with vitality and comfort, and it all begins with the nourishment you provide your body. Cheers to a healthier tomorrow and a more vibrant you!

MEAL

TRACKER

Monday	Breakfast	Lunch	Dinner

Tuesday	Breakfast	Lunch	Dinner

Wednesday	Breakfast	Lunch	Dinner

Thursday	Breakfast	Lunch	Dinner

Friday	Breakfast	Lunch	Dinner

Saturday	Breakfast	Lunch	Dinner

Sunday	Breakfast	Lunch	Dinner

<table>
<tr><td rowspan="2">Monday</td><td>Breakfast</td><td>Lunch</td><td>Dinner</td></tr>
<tr><td></td><td></td><td></td></tr>
</table>

<table>
<tr><td rowspan="2">Tuesday</td><td>Breakfast</td><td>Lunch</td><td>Dinner</td></tr>
<tr><td></td><td></td><td></td></tr>
</table>

<table>
<tr><td rowspan="2">Wednesday</td><td>Breakfast</td><td>Lunch</td><td>Dinner</td></tr>
<tr><td></td><td></td><td></td></tr>
</table>

<table>
<tr><td rowspan="2">Thursday</td><td>Breakfast</td><td>Lunch</td><td>Dinner</td></tr>
<tr><td></td><td></td><td></td></tr>
</table>

<table>
<tr><td rowspan="2">Friday</td><td>Breakfast</td><td>Lunch</td><td>Dinner</td></tr>
<tr><td></td><td></td><td></td></tr>
</table>

<table>
<tr><td rowspan="2">Saturday</td><td>Breakfast</td><td>Lunch</td><td>Dinner</td></tr>
<tr><td></td><td></td><td></td></tr>
</table>

<table>
<tr><td rowspan="2">Sunday</td><td>Breakfast</td><td>Lunch</td><td>Dinner</td></tr>
<tr><td></td><td></td><td></td></tr>
</table>

	Breakfast	Lunch	Dinner
Monday			

	Breakfast	Lunch	Dinner
Tuesday			

	Breakfast	Lunch	Dinner
Wednesday			

	Breakfast	Lunch	Dinner
Thursday			

	Breakfast	Lunch	Dinner
Friday			

	Breakfast	Lunch	Dinner
Saturday			

	Breakfast	Lunch	Dinner
Sunday			

Monday	Breakfast	Lunch	Dinner

Tuesday	Breakfast	Lunch	Dinner

Wednesday	Breakfast	Lunch	Dinner

Thursday	Breakfast	Lunch	Dinner

Friday	Breakfast	Lunch	Dinner

Saturday	Breakfast	Lunch	Dinner

Sunday	Breakfast	Lunch	Dinner

Monday	Breakfast	Lunch	Dinner

Tuesday	Breakfast	Lunch	Dinner

Wednesday	Breakfast	Lunch	Dinner

Thursday	Breakfast	Lunch	Dinner

Friday	Breakfast	Lunch	Dinner

Saturday	Breakfast	Lunch	Dinner

Sunday	Breakfast	Lunch	Dinner

	Breakfast	Lunch	Dinner
Monday			
Tuesday			
Wednesday			
Thursday			
Friday			
Saturday			
Sunday			

Monday	Breakfast	Lunch	Dinner

Tuesday	Breakfast	Lunch	Dinner

Wednesday	Breakfast	Lunch	Dinner

Thursday	Breakfast	Lunch	Dinner

Friday	Breakfast	Lunch	Dinner

Saturday	Breakfast	Lunch	Dinner

Sunday	Breakfast	Lunch	Dinner

Monday	Breakfast	Lunch	Dinner

Tuesday	Breakfast	Lunch	Dinner

Wednesday	Breakfast	Lunch	Dinner

Thursday	Breakfast	Lunch	Dinner

Friday	Breakfast	Lunch	Dinner

Saturday	Breakfast	Lunch	Dinner

Sunday	Breakfast	Lunch	Dinner

Monday	Breakfast	Lunch	Dinner

Tuesday	Breakfast	Lunch	Dinner

Wednesday	Breakfast	Lunch	Dinner

Thursday	Breakfast	Lunch	Dinner

Friday	Breakfast	Lunch	Dinner

Saturday	Breakfast	Lunch	Dinner

Sunday	Breakfast	Lunch	Dinner

<table>
<tr><td rowspan="2">Monday</td><td>Breakfast</td><td>Lunch</td><td>Dinner</td></tr>
<tr><td></td><td></td><td></td></tr>
</table>

<table>
<tr><td rowspan="2">Tuesday</td><td>Breakfast</td><td>Lunch</td><td>Dinner</td></tr>
<tr><td></td><td></td><td></td></tr>
</table>

<table>
<tr><td rowspan="2">Wednesday</td><td>Breakfast</td><td>Lunch</td><td>Dinner</td></tr>
<tr><td></td><td></td><td></td></tr>
</table>

<table>
<tr><td rowspan="2">Thursday</td><td>Breakfast</td><td>Lunch</td><td>Dinner</td></tr>
<tr><td></td><td></td><td></td></tr>
</table>

<table>
<tr><td rowspan="2">Friday</td><td>Breakfast</td><td>Lunch</td><td>Dinner</td></tr>
<tr><td></td><td></td><td></td></tr>
</table>

<table>
<tr><td rowspan="2">Saturday</td><td>Breakfast</td><td>Lunch</td><td>Dinner</td></tr>
<tr><td></td><td></td><td></td></tr>
</table>

<table>
<tr><td rowspan="2">Sunday</td><td>Breakfast</td><td>Lunch</td><td>Dinner</td></tr>
<tr><td></td><td></td><td></td></tr>
</table>